Sex Position Secrets

Sexy games with Kama-sutra positions. Lean how easy you can have an orgasm and discover the best tantric positions

by

Scarlett Hunter

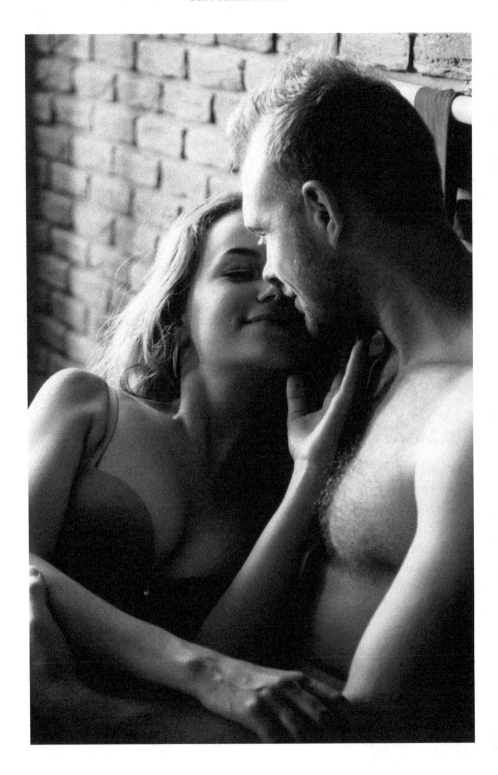

Table of Contents

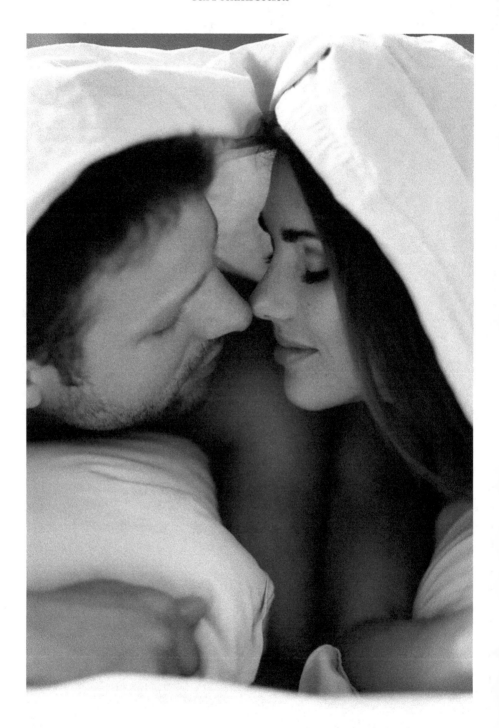

Introduction

There is much more to the Kama Sutra than just sex positions, and this book is aimed at teaching you everything it has to offer. From the art of seduction and flirting, to how to choose a spouse, this book will start at the very beginning before it delves deeper into the art of sex.

While topics like courtship may differ from how we do things today, there is still an underlying truth to all aspects. Whether we are meeting lovers in 2nd century India, at a bar, or via a dating app, the basic concepts remain unchanged, as we are all striving for the same outcome — attraction and romance.

Some may think that this book has very little to offer since it was written so long ago, but you will be amazed at how relevant the Kama Sutra still is today. Not only does it discuss the art of sex itself, but it showcases how you can elevate your sex life from a boring routine into something mind-blowing.

Beyond just the sexual aspects, it also offers advice on how to treat your lover, before, during, and after sex. It is about how to connect with a person, how to pleasure them, and even how to make them your spouse.

There is so much more to sex than just the act itself, and we hope to cover everything for you so that you are fully equipped to enhance your sex life and be the best lover you can be.

The history of the Kama Sutra is rich with information, and it is a fascinating look at how love and intimacy were once regarded, as well as how it is still applicable today. There is a reason that the Kama Sutra is still read by many people to this day, regardless of how long ago it was written.

There are plenty of books on this subject on the market, thanks again for choosing this one! Every effort was made to ensure it is full of as much useful information as possible. Please enjoy!

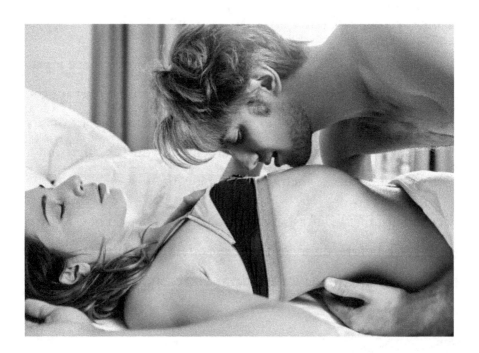

Chapter 1:

Positions to Try out

It's enticing to take off your clothing and go on when you have strong sexual interaction with someone. But it is a great pleasure to take time to sample the encounter. You can feel more relaxed, linked, and stimulated if you involve your body and mind in your interaction, resulting in better sex.

By taking your time and being imaginative, you can also avoid the risk of making a repetitive sex with the same steps, in the same place, having the same result.

This chapter aims to bring you some fresh ideas with which to play in the bedroom and new positions that you may not have tried, which will offer you more pleasure. Nonetheless, new positions alone won't mean great sex. To make everything perfect, use those tips and make your love more alive.

Before Sex

As we have already mentioned in the previous chapters of this book, sexual arousal can begin many hours before the encounter itself.

And indeed, it is good to make this happen. Wondering how?

There is no standard procedure, but the secret lies in generating a desire, in teasing the mind of your partner.

It can be something said in the morning before you part, a phone call or a text sent during the day, or even sending sensual photos.

What can be said has a wide range of choices; for example, it can be a simple "what would you like to do to me," or "what would I do to you," a sensual memory, a dirty proposal, etc.

In this way, you will create a fixed thought in your partner's mind, which will increase the desired moment by moment until you are finally together.

The next step can be a romantic dinner, whether in a restaurant or at home, where you could continue to tease your partner's mind with allusions, or caresses hidden under the table.

The icing on the cake could be having your bedroom set up romantically, or making sure it is at least clean, tidy and smelling good!

And finally, even sexy lingerie makes a good impression.

You are now ready to begin your foreplay.

During Sex

To make the experience as pleasant and unforgettable as possible, it is necessary to proceed slowly, and let there be a constant crescendo of emotions and sensations before orgasm.

First, you have to create a strong intimacy, a connection, an emotional involvement for both of you.

Go ahead for intense looks, kisses and simple caresses, even before undressing.

Even exchanging some exciting little words could be beneficial, you could say, for example, how much you have desired each other. At this point, use all the notions you have learned about foreplay, remembering that the genitals must be the last area to be included in the game.

Once you get to the height of desire, you are finally ready to try some new position.

The advice is to try more than one in single sexual intercourse, in order to prolong the session even more, and consequently, prolong the pleasure.

Before reaching orgasm, stop and change your position. And so on, until the moment arrives when you can no longer wait, the desire is sky high, the enjoyment is pure, and you just have to welcome the great O.

Positions that give you a complete picture of each other's naked bodies may produce arousals so soon, while those that make eye contact improve intimacy and tend to make the enjoyment more slowly. Make sure to don't insist on a position that creates discomfort for one of you; you would risk ruining the moment; rather, go straight to the next choice.

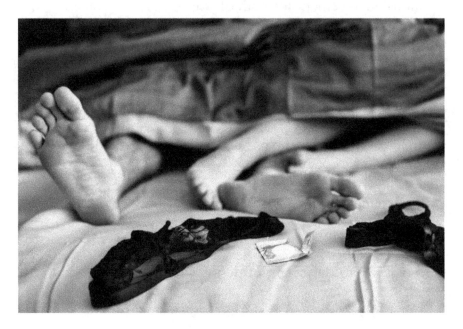

The woman on the top

As we already said, the woman on top position is good for relaxation and stimulation of the G-spot.

The location of the female on the top helps you to have a visual contact and offers the advantage of being able to control the speed and extent of penetration. In fact, the deepest penetration is not always to be assumed as the best option. The sex therapist Rebecca

Rosenblatt has written in her book Seducing Your Man:' Shallow will stimulate the front third of the vagina, which is the most sensitive.

Hot tip — When a man stimulates a woman manually or orally until she is extremely excited, it's simpler to climax her. So let her squat on the head from the woman-on-top role to motivate her orally.

The Cowgirl

With the man lying on his back, the woman straddles her hips and position herself over his penis. Smearing it with some lube beforehand will add to your pleasure. She can hold his erect penis in one hand and slide down onto it.

The key element of this position is not to sit upright on top of him, but to lean forward over him, which means the woman can use her hands to support herself, either placing them on his hips, or either on the side of him.

Once in the position, she can swivel her hips like a dancer, bounce or grind on him and control the depth and rhythm of your thrusts.

If the woman like some really deep penetration, she can move into a more upright position, and she could also try spreading her knees further apart. Additionally, the man can put their hands on her hips for extra leverage and to maximize the impact of the grind.

Reverse Cowgirl a.k.a. Rodeo Drive

One of the best things about the Reverse Cowgirl position that makes it easier for those who are a little shy or nervous being on top is that the woman doesn't have to face her man while performing it, which takes a lot of the 'performance pressure' or anxiety out of the equation that some girls feel when on top of their man. Note that the Reverse Cowgirl is perfect for anal sex as well as regular vaginal sex.

The man lies on his back with his legs outstretched. The woman straddles him with her butt toward him. The woman then lowers herself onto his penis completely before getting down on her knees. Then she can lean forward and press her hands into his legs, moving her butt up and down as gently or as vigorously as she wants, or maybe she can just grind on him.

She can also try to change the angle of entry leaning backward, using her hands as support, and see how it feels.

When leaning backward, the man can also use his arms to give better support.

During the reverse cowgirl, the man can choose either to have a passive or an active role. If he wants to become more involved, then he can grind back up against her, as she is grinding on him, or he can thrust up and down.

There are many variations for this position, for example:

- Reverse Asian cowgirl: This time, the woman will have her knees raised up, squatting up and down on him. In this position, she has all the control, while her body is wide open for her man to enjoy visually. He will also have the pleasure of watching her going up and down on his penis.

- Titanic: In this position, the man's legs are slightly bent at the knees and feet are fixed on the surface. The woman's legs are bent in knees and laid along his buttocks. She gently sinks the thighs around the man. Her hands are outstretched forward and located on man's knees to make support. Her belly is tightly pressed against his hips. She slightly leans her head backward.

- Or you can also switch roles by performing the Reverse Cowboy sex position, where the man is on top, straddling her and bending his penis right down to enter. To perform this, you need to make sure that the man has lots of penile flexibility!

Seated

The love seat

The love seat position is a great chance for couples who usually just have sex when lying down or in bed. You can use the Back Seat Driver practically anywhere in your house, in the bedroom, living room, kitchen, etc.

In fact, the love seat sex position is a seated position that uses a chair or other sturdy piece of furniture for support. To get into the position, the man will be sitting on the edge of a chair, a sofa, or even the bed with his legs spread wide and his feet on the floor. The woman can either then climb onto his lap for a face to face position or back up onto the man's crotch and let him slowly slide his penis inside while bending her knees.

In this position, the woman will be doing most of the work, bouncing up and down on the man. She can also hold onto the man's shoulders or the back of the chair to help them move and thrust.

You can vary the depth of penetration in the love seat position by having the man adjust their position on the chair; sitting closer to the edge should provide more depth.

The Lap Dance

The Lap Dance position is a sex position very similar to the love seat and where the man can relax and 'enjoy the show' just like he would in a strip club, but he also has the option of being a bit more active.

You can probably guess that the Lap Dance is mostly about the man's pleasure. So keep this in mind when performing it. To start, the man needs to sit down on a comfortable sofa or seat.

The woman can, at this point, have a little bit of a Striptease show before approaching him. She can ask him to kiss her nipples and explore all the erogenous zones while exhibiting.

When both ready, the woman will be on her feet and will back up onto the man. She can grab his penis and guide it into her vagina.

Once he is inside, she can lean forwards or backward on him, depending on how intimate you want to make it. Then she can slowly grind on him while he stays deep inside. (This can provide fantastic G-Spot stimulation).

Or she can bounce up and down on him. Be mind that leaning forward will be easier for bouncing while leaning backward is better for grinding.

Side by Side

Traditional Spooning

Sweet and romantic, this position is ideal for those who love to cuddle.

Both man and woman lie on their sides with the man snuggled close to his lady's back. She draws her legs into her chest, allowing for an easy penetration from behind. Her lover can use his hands to caress her from the front.

Once everything starts to get hotter, the woman can make it more exciting by getting frisky with her legs: she can lift one up toward the ceiling, bend one and place her foot on top of the other shin, bend both knees drastically. All of these twists will change the feeling of fullness inside her.

This is an ideal position if you have a knee injury or if you are pregnant, as it keeps the weight away from your body. The man can stretch his legs out straight or spoon them into his lady's legs.

Spoon Facing a.k.a Sidewinder

The facing spoon sex position is a sex position in which couples lie on their sides and face each other. The woman then spreads her legs slightly and the man enters her. Once his penis is inside her vagina, she can then put her legs back together, putting her clitoris in a position to be stimulated by the shaft of his penis.

Having sex in this position can be much more intimate than the traditional intercourse. It's much easier for a couple to kiss, hug and caress.

However, it can be somewhat tricky for a man to thrust in and out of a woman's vagina in this position, so couples may need to get a little creative. For instance, instead of traditional thrusting, couples can try grinding together or moving their pelvises in circular motions to enhance the pleasure.

Warming Tip: Hug each other for a while before you get active. Hugging elevates the oxytocin levels, which produce a bonding compound, which will strengthen the connection.

Spoon and fork combo, a.k.a. spork

This sex position is a twist of the spooning position and was so-named because the woman's legs take the form of a fork and a spoon.

This is another sex position that makes couples look forward to the next time they are having sex. Pulling it off is quite easy because it involves the woman lying on her back and spreading her legs.

The man will then lie across and opposite her in a 90-degree position, thus getting to hit it directly from below.

This time the man gets to take the reins, and he'll be rewarded with an awesome view of the woman's body. This position is also great because the woman is free to do with her hands as she pleases. She can either play with her boobs or clitoris, depending on whatever she prefers. A little exchange of dirty talk and eye contact can go a long way in lighting things up a bit.

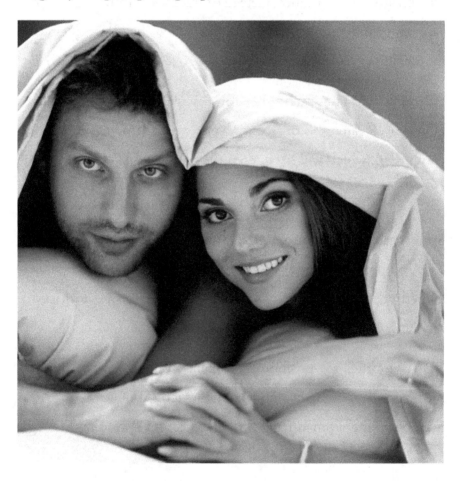

Head to Toe

The Spider, a.k.a. The Crab Walk

The Spider position begins with the couple facing each other, both in a seated position. The woman is the first to lie back while the man scoots in between her legs, achieving penetration.

Next, it's the man's turn to lie back, being careful to maintain his erection inside her. If the couple is in the position correctly, each partner should be lying flat on their back with their head in between the other's legs, buttocks touching.

To improve the possibility of greater movement, the couple can bring both knees up so that they each have something to grip during the motions. The couple is now instructed to wiggle, gyrate, and grind their buttocks anyway they like.

Snow Angel a.k.a. Bottom's Up

The Snow angel sex position comes in to save adults' sex life from running cold. The woman lies on her back with her legs open, and the man lies on top of her with his head face down by her legs and the butt toward her face.

She lifts her legs and wraps them around his back to elevate her pelvis for deep penetration. He spreads his legs to the sides, revealing an amazing rear view. She can then grab his butt to help him slide up and back. She can add a little massage action to her grip also. Or she can eventually tease his most erogenous zones like anus or testes.

Crisscross or the X Position

The crisscross is a very exotic looking but fairly easy to perform sex position.

To perform the crisscross sex position, the woman starts by lying on her side so that one leg is on the bed and the other leg is raised and bent right on top of it. The man is also going to be lying on his side.

But he will be lying so that his head is close to her feet. He now needs to slip his lower leg underneath her lower leg right by her crotch. Next, he will put his upper leg over her lower leg and move his crotch towards until he can penetrate.

So the woman's lower leg will be between the man legs. After he enters, he just needs to start thrusting. The woman just needs to 'go with the flow' of the man. In other words, she can gently thrust back onto the man as he is thrusting into her.

This position might not allow much range of motion, but don't be discouraged — there's plenty of pleasure to be had for all! The positioning of your intertwined legs provides the woman a continuous clitoral stimulation, while the shallow thrusts excite the nerve endings on the head of his penis, allowing for an electrifying build to orgasm.

Oral Stimulation

The Bees Knees

Most couples consider this position to be among the best sex positions, and it is so for a number of reasons. First, the position has everything to do with wet, sensual fellatio, something both men and women can't resist. This sex position involves the woman sucking her man off while on his knees.

Once she's comfortable, the man can put his throbbing penis into her mouth and she can suck him for as long as possible. This position also allows the woman to play with her man's butt, balls, and abs.

The man, on the other hand, can run his fingers through her hair while whispering sweet, erotic words into her ears. The bee's knees sex position is also convenient for maintaining strong eye contact. Nothing makes a man happier than looking down at the girl of his dreams, sucking him off in this position.

When the man finally reaches orgasm and the moment of ejaculation arrives, the woman can decide whether to let him come into her mouth and taste his semen or whether to direct the penis elsewhere, on her breasts, for example.

Also, to ensure the woman doesn't end up bruising her knees, finding something soft and comfortable for her to kneel on should always be prioritized.

69 and Inverted 69

A 69 is the act of two people simultaneously giving each other oral sex. During a 69 position, one person is stretched, lying on the back, while the other is on top, face down and with his head pointing at the other person's genitals so that the mouths of the two people point to each one's genitals at the same time.

Traditional 69 wants women staying on the top while for the inverted 69 is the man staying on top. In this case, the man has to be careful to properly bent his knees in the way that his penis is in the right position above the woman's mouth.

There are also other variations for the 69 position; some are simple, while others may require more physical effort.

A simple one can be the sideways 69 in which Instead of positioning one on top of the other, both participants are lying on their sides.

Or also the squatting 69 in which the man is seated while the woman back on him bent over, reaching his genital with her face and having her butt toward his face. While on of the most challenging ones can be the standing 69, in which the man stands and holds up the woman upside down, high enough to lead her face to his penis, and to be able to mouth her vagina.

Sensorial Tip— Place on your bedside a cup of warm tea and an ice cube. Alternate the ice cube and the drink in your mouth while giving oral sex.

A butterfly hover a.k.a. The Face Sitter

Face-Sitting is an oral sex position that will be approached by you and your partner from totally different perspectives. One person lays down and positions their face directly under the genitals of their partner, who is hovering from above, and performs oral sex.

The partner receiving should gently kneel over their partner's face, with their head directly between their legs. Once you're sitting, feel free to change directions (it's fun to switch it up!) and tell your partner what feels good.

This position is mostly used with a woman sitting on top, as the man. Contrariwise is very hard from this position to do a full blow job, so it could mainly be only testes oral stimulation.

Anal sex

Despite the possibilities of pure enjoyment, it can give, whether it is for religious reasons, physical or psychological discomfort, or a matter of hygiene, anal intercourse is a hard topic to deal with.

So let's break a few myths and explore how to think about anal sex before you can start a safe conversation with your partner about bringing anal sex into your relationship.

Anal sex is gross. Anal sex is filthy. Although there is a room of germs, this problem can be easily overcome in two ways:

- An anal bath: The best way to clean your ass prior to anal sex is with a water enema. Starting at the drugstore, purchase yourself a standard water enema kit. This should include a hot water bottle, a hose, a plug and a rectal tip.

When you bring your kit home, fill the hot water bottle with water until it is roughly 90 percent full.

Then, close the bottle with the plug, fasten the hose to the plug (making sure the clamp on the hose is closer toward the bottom and closed), and finally, attach the rectal tip to the bottom of the hose. You might want to coat the tip in some lubricant to assist in insertion.

Then, lay down in the tub and insert the rectal tip into your butt and open the clamp. If the water pressure is too strong, close the clamp, wait, re-open it and let the water work its way through you until the hot water bottle is empty.

When empty, the objective here is to keep the water in your body for as long as you can. Three to 15 minutes is great, but this all depends on how often you've done this. When the water is in your body, rotate to help coat the entire colon in water. Then, empty yourself into the toilet.

- Using condoms: Condoms are the best way of protection from bacterial and viral infections. And they can also shield from the dirt inside the rectum.

As for physical pain, this can certainly be avoided through the use of a good silicone lubricant, the use of sphincter relaxation techniques, and communication and collaboration between partners.

Another bad myth to be disproved is the belief that male anal sex is only for homosexuals.

Be sure anal playing isn't homosexual; it is just erotic.

Wheatear, you are a man or a woman; if you never had anal sex is worthy to give it a try.

Some people really adore anal sex. They find it incredibly pleasurable, while others don't find it pleasurable at all. It comes down to personal preference, so if you try it and don't enjoy it, that's fine. There's no need to stress about it if you don't get much stimulation from it.

Having made these considerations and bringing to mind all the notions learned in the previous chapters regarding the anatomy of the rectum, we can now explore the best ways to prepare for anal sex, and the best positions to perform.

Set the stage

Before it all begins, it's good to prepare yourself physically and psychologically.

So go ahead and take care of your hygiene, you can wash yourself thoroughly or take an anal bath if it makes you feel better.

Make sure you have enough lube, condoms and wipes, and if you like, some sex toys too. You might be tempted to search for a product that numbs your anus for anal sex. However, these products aren't lubricants and prevent you from knowing what is happening with your body. You could potentially be numb when a serious tear has occurred, and numbing ingredients may also be irritants.

If this is your first time, it would be good to venture into some self-stimulation so that you get used to the sensation.

During anal sex, there can be a lot of tension, and you will need a lot of communication with your partner to make sure that the experience is as enjoyable for both of you, and that there are no complications.

So make sure you create the right intimacy and relaxation before starting.

It wouldn't be a bad idea to start with regular foreplay, to release tension and spark arousal.

Warm up: Rub Them the Right Way for Trust and Relaxation
Now I will explain to you the best technique to prepare the anus to penetration. To make the description simpler, we assume that you, the reader, are the woman who is to be penetrated by your man.

To start with, your partner needs to apply a bit lube to the tip of his finger and some more to your anus. Next, he needs to slowly slide his finger inside you, millimeter by millimeter, while you give him feedback, telling him if to go deeper or to stop moving or to SLOWLY pull out (pulling out fast can cause some pain, he needs to do it very slowly).

As he softly penetrates you deeper and deeper with his finger, you should feel it reasonably comfortable. If it becomes slightly uncomfortable, then tell him to stop moving and to keep his finger still for a minute or two. This will allow your sphincter to relax around his finger and open up. When the pain subsides, he can push a little deeper. If it becomes too uncomfortable and painful, again then tell him to pull his finger out slowly. Rest for a minute or two and then get him to start over.

Once he can't penetrate you any deeper with his finger, he needs to slowly thrust in and out. Again you should control the pace here, so tell to him either speed up or slow down, depending on what you feel and like.

When you are comfortable with your partner thrusting in and out, he needs to try adding a second finger. Again, he should be very slow and cautious doing this, following your instructions and feedback to either continue, slow down, stop or slowly pull out. (Also, make sure there is still plenty of lube!) Once he can easily thrust in and out with his two fingers, then either try three fingers, then you can start having anal sex.

The most comfortable position to start having anal sex is with your man on his back so that you are in control. This means that it's a lot harder for him to thrust into you, and it's much easier for you to control how deep you take him and how fast he thrusts.

So get him to lie down on his back and ask him NOT to thrust into you. Instead, he should remain still. After applying some lube to your man and your backside, you can then straddle him on your knees like in the Cowgirl position or even the Asian Cowgirl position.

Grab hold of his penis and then slowly guide it inside your anus. Make sure to take your time. As mentioned above, if you feel uncomfortable or experience any type of pain, stop and allow your sphincter muscle to relax around his cock. Once it has, then you can try taking him a little deeper.

When your man is completely inside you and can't go any deeper, you can slowly raise your body up and down. The main thing here is again to take things slowly. You don't want to hurt yourself, so if you experience any discomfort at all, slow right down and even stop to allow yourself to relax.

Once you do feel comfortable moving up and down on your man, then he can start to get involved a little more by thrusting himself. Remember that you still need to be in control here. So if he gets too carried away, tell him to slow down or stop.

Training

If you rarely have anal sex, your sphincter never gets used to relaxing for your man's penis. This means that each time you have anal sex, it feels like the first time for your sphincter and it never learns to relax fully and open up. The only way to overcome this is to have anal sex regularly.

Once you have tried anal sex with your man a few times, you'll start to notice that your sphincter relaxes more rapidly and that having anal sex becomes more and more enjoyable for you.

When this starts happening, then you need to start doing some experimentation so that you learn how to get maximum pleasure from anal, and the try new positions

You can try:

- Experiment with short, shallow strokes as well as long, deep, penetrating strokes to see what you prefer.
- Experiment with different angles. Does a particular angle feel better than the rest? Does a little experimentation to see what you prefer?

Once you are comfortable with your man having more control and doing all the thrusting, then you may want to try out some new position.

It could be a doggy style or spooning type positions, where your man is penetrating you from behind, or if you rather have some eye contact, you can try some missionary style position, with your butt up.

Finally, once you have gained enough experience, you can start thinking about adding new stimuli, such as double penetration, with the help of a dildo or a vibrator.

At this point make sure not to do any kind of double dipping, since, as we have already mentioned in the previous chapters, switching from anal sex to vaginal sex without changing condoms and thoroughly cleaning the penis or sex toy is going to lead to an infection.

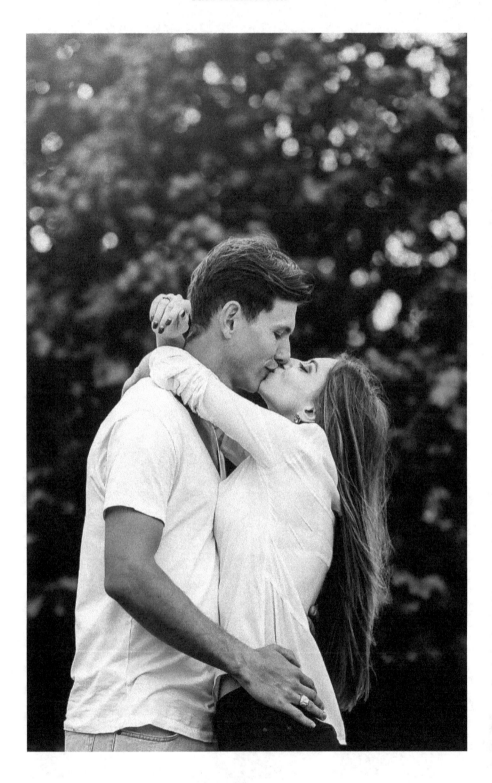

Chapter 2:

What is the Kama Sutra

I t is unlikely that you have never heard of the Kama Sutra before, but you may be unfamiliar with what exactly it is. Some may think of it as simply a book of sex positions, while others may know a bit more of the history and how it came to be.

This chapter will look at the history behind the Kama Sutra, discussing the literal meaning of the words, as well as what it teaches us, and how it is meant to be used. Since the Kama Sutra originated in India, there are also many terms and words used throughout that you may not be familiar with, so we will make sure to breakdown some of the most commonly seen ones and provide their definitions.

With such a rich history behind it, there is so much to learn about the Kama Sutra. It is an expansive work of literature that was created to be more than just a guide on different ways in which you can have sex.

Instead, it permeates all aspects of life and brings together both sexual and non-sexual ways in which you interact with a lover, a partner, or a spouse. But what exactly does "Kama Sutra" mean?

Meaning Behind the Name

The word "Kama" is one that means pleasure but can also be translated as desire or longing. There is a sexual connotation associated with the word, meaning it is more to do with sexual pleasure and desire than with the pleasures of life or desire for material goods, but that doesn't mean that the Kama Sutra as a whole is limited to only sexual pleasure. "Sutra," on the other hand, translates to verse or scripture.

When you put these words together, you get the translation of "Scripture of Pleasure," but there are many variations on how you can literally translate this.

Delving deeper into the meaning behind the name, the pleasure that is Kama is one that is of all five senses, and this is very important. While many think of the Kama Sutra as a sex book, it is actually a book that focuses on pleasing all of the senses and is meant to be a guide on how to live a good life and enjoy yourself.

From the physical enjoyment of sex to the pleasure that is derived from being in love, the Kama Sutra is filled with different verses that cover a wide range of different activities and pleasures.

While we did mention that Kama often has a sexual connotation, like with all translations, there are different meanings depending on how it is being used. Kama can also be used when referencing love or affection, and in this sense, it is used in a non-sexual way.

This is why the Kama Sutra needs to be viewed as a whole since it was not intended to simply be a sexual book, but more so an erotic manual on life.

We know that the Kama Sutra extends beyond just the physical pleasures, as the book touches on the four different virtues of life. Those four are:

- **Dharma** – How to live a virtuous life

- **Kama** – How to enjoy the pleasures of the senses

- **Moksha** – How to be liberated from the cycle of reincarnation

- **Artha** – How to gain material wealth

These four virtues are tenants of Hinduism, which is applicable since the Kama Sutra originates in India where Hinduism is one of the predominant religions.

This historical context allows us to understand the book better, as we need to approach it from the mindset of the author, who would have most likely been a practicing Hindu.

The author saw sexual pleasure as one of the main virtues of life, and it was both a necessary and spiritual pursuit that was important both from a non-sexual and sexual avenue. These virtues are almost instructions on how a person should live in order to be fulfilled both in this life as well as in the afterlife.

Regardless of what your personal religion is, all the points are still applicable, as basic human nature dictates that we are all attempting to be the best version of ourselves and to accomplish everything we set out to gain. Some other words that you may encounter within the Kama Sutra, and their translations, are:

- **Devi** – Goddess

- **Gandharva** – A form of marriage in which everyone is consenting to it

- **Lingam** – Penis

- **Nayika** – A woman who is desired by someone

- **Prahanana** – Striking or slapping someone during sex

- **Raja** – King

- **Shlokas** – Messages from above that are used to end every chapter of the Kama Sutra

- **Vatsala** – A married woman who has children

- **Vikrant** – A brave and beloved man

- **Yoni** – Vagina

Within this book, we will try and use as much of the original language as possible, so having a glossary of terms will be beneficial.

With that said, however, there will always be translations available throughout so that you can follow along with ease.

So why does the literal meaning of the name even matter?

Well, understanding what an author is trying to convey is important as it allows us to enter the book and adjust our personal views so that we do not bring in our biases and preconceived notions.

If you come into the Kama Sutra thinking it should only include some sex positions and nothing more, then you miss out on the richness that is contained within.

Likewise, if you ignore the historical significance behind the text, you fail to grasp many of the concepts located within.

In order to gain as much as you can from the Kama Sutra, you need to know what the author intended with it, and why they felt the need to create this work of literature.

To assist you in this goal, we will delve further into the history and intention later in this chapter.

History of the Kama Sutra

The exact date that the Kama Sutra was written is not known, but estimates place it anywhere between 400 BCE and 300 CE. What we do know, however, is that it was officially compiled and turned into the book that we know today in the 2nd century, otherwise known as 2 CE.

This does not mean though that the book has not undergone revisions since then, and some scholars believe that the version we have is actually closely linked to the 3rd century, as some of the references throughout would not have been applicable to the 2nd century.

With the text being so old, exact dating is virtually impossible; nevertheless, there is a lot of information we do know about it.

We do know that the text originates from India, although the exact location is unknown.

Historians have been able to narrow down the location to somewhere within the north or northwest region but beyond that, it is a guess as to where the author was from.

As for the author himself, we do know it was written by a man named Vatsyayana Mallanaga, as his name is engraved into the beginning of the text. Who this man was is unclear, but we do have information as to why he wrote the Kama Sutra?

Since it's compilation in the 2nd-3rd century, the Kama Sutra has undergone numerous translations and there are versions in almost every language. It was originally written in Sanskrit, an ancient Indian language, and this is the language that many Hindu scriptures were written in.

While some translations are quite accurate, it is important to note that some translators did place their own bias into their work, and that can be seen in the discrepancies that were later found. One of the key examples of this was in the 19th century when the Kama Sutra was translated into English.

The translator at that time wanted to ensure that the role of women in the sexual realm was not as prominent, as that was not the culture of the times.

In order to maintain that societal understanding of sex and women, the Kama Sutra was altered so that women were significantly downplayed throughout. This has since been corrected, but it is important to be aware of this if you ever decide to pick up a copy for yourself as you want to be sure you are getting a purer translation.

The foundations of the Kama Sutra are rooted within the Vedic Era of literature, which is based on the word Vedas. Vedas were historical texts written in India around this time that dealt with lifestyle and how one should conduct themselves on a daily basis.

All works of this time period were verbally passed down, and traditions were later adapted into many of the Hindu beliefs that are now practiced today. In the Vedic Era, there were distinct classes and castes within society, and a lot of that is reflected within the Kama Sutra.

Many references are made to those who are in differing classes, and how relationships between individuals of different castes cannot work out. While this type of information is not apparently meaningful in today's culture, it does cross over when we look at socio-economic statuses and how the rich and poor interact even today.

These foundations are incredibly important because they shape the mind frame of the author of the Kama Sutra. Without grasping the history, you cannot possibly grasp what is being discussed, as many of the terms and concepts no longer exist or are practiced currently.

It is with this in mind that we can start to see that the Kama Sutra is a religious text by some accounts. We may not associate sex and religion as being intertwined, but in fact, Vatsyayana saw sex as being a religious experience as well as a requirement to live a proper life.

The basis of the entire viewpoint stems from certain religious beliefs, and the foundation for the entire book comes from his personal, religious beliefs. It is a celebration of human sexuality and the most carnal of pleasures, which are gifts from the gods and ultimately a necessity in life.

Philosophy of the Kama Sutra

As we said, we do know a bit about why Vatsyayana wrote the Kama Sutra. Looking at ancient Hindu texts, we know that the four virtues were commonly discussed and written at length about.

Many of the texts focused on the two important virtues of Dharma (morality), and Athra (prosperity), while few really delved into the importance of Kama (pleasure).

Vatsyayana meditated upon this reality and came to the conclusion that Kama was just as important as all of the other virtues, and so it was only proper to have a guide written solely about how to obtain Kama.

The four virtues can be looked at more like goals that each person much work towards within their lifetime in order to lead a complete and fulfilled life.

Within the Kama Sutra, there are many references to the other virtues as they are all tied together and must be achieved in order to succeed. One cannot simply focus on the physical pleasures and ignore the need for morality or prosperity, so you may notice throughout that sex and morality are often combined, as well as sex and finding a partner that brings about monetary prosperity.

To understand the philosophy behind the Kama Sutra, it is vital that you understand what it was intended to be. The sex acts that are described throughout are little more than theatrics, with an emphasis on outrageous and yoga-inspired poses.

The goal was unlikely to be used as a literal manual, but instead to be used as a way to understand both society and the individual.

A vast majority of the book is taken up by discussing how men and women interact within society, both as a whole and simply with each other. It can be seen as almost a screenplay, taking us on a journey of love within ancient Indian times.

There is talk of love, intimacy, and mundane tasks such as bathing and grooming. The Kama Sutra is a manual on all aspects of pleasure, both in the sexual sense and in the day to day realm.

Kama is so often seen as something that is less important than other aspects of human pursuit. We are told to work hard, earn money, find a spouse, have children, and live a moral and righteous life.

But rarely are advised on how to let loose and enjoy ourselves, or how important of a role sex plays in the human experience.

The Kama Sutra is the bridge over that gap, intended to lift up the importance of pleasure and sex, and place it in as high of regard as all the other aspects we are expected to work towards.

Some have questioned whether or not the Kama Sutra really is a female positive as it may appear, but if you approach it from the idea of the times, then it can actually be seen as more of a feminist work of art than the surface would suggest.

There is an obvious sexual freedom that is discussed within, one in which even our current societal viewpoint doesn't always acknowledge. Try bringing up the topic of female masturbation and see the sudden puritanical viewpoint that many people rush to.

Movies are quick to showcase men in a sexual manner, but female sexuality is much more often subdued or removed completely from the narrative. To have a book that explores the different facets of a woman's sexuality is unique both historically as well as in the current climate.

Given that the Kama Sutra talks almost nothing of procreation, it truly highlights the idea that this is a guide for pleasure and nothing more. So, by its own very nature, it is also a book dedicated to a woman's pleasure, both by herself and that which is given to her by her partner.

Beyond just sex, the Kama Sutra also discusses how to treat a woman properly so that she is nurtured and cared for in all aspects of life. It discusses showering her with affection and gifts and giving her absolute power when it comes to the home's finances.

From a philosophical standpoint, the Kama Sutra opens our minds to the needs of both men and women, and it does a good job of including women in the discussion, especially for the times.

Not only does it take a more liberal and open-minded approach to women, but that same approach is extended to homosexuality and bisexuality as well. There are many references and discussions about men sleeping with men, and women pleasuring other women, as well as advice on having threesomes and even orgies.

Whatever the sexual desire is of the individual is both encouraged and celebrated, and there is no judgment cast upon those who may differ from what is considered the norm.

The Kama Sutra makes us think by challenging our conceptions and internalized beliefs when it comes to sex. Whether it is something we partake in or not, it opens our eyes to the different forms of relationships that can exist both romantically and sexually and offers up advice on how to succeed in achieving absolute pleasure.

It removes the idea that sex should be for procreating and instead emphasizes the pleasure that can be found within a sexual encounter.

On a deeper level, it challenges the notion that physical pleasure should take a backseat to otherworldly pursuits, and that pleasure is just as important in life as everything else. For a life without pleasure, it isn't truly a life worth living at all.

What Does it Teach Us?

The Kama Sutra teaches us many things, from how to take care of ourselves, to how to take care of our partner. Everything begins with you, and how you groom yourself and carry yourself in this world.

It is an extremely practical guide that mixes real-world advice with philosophical ideas and concepts. It is meant to make us sit back and think about why we do what we do and how we can live a better life overall. But all of that begins with the individual person.

Even if we only look at the sexual aspect of the Kama Sutra, we can see exactly what the author is attempting to teach us about physical pleasure. None of us would exist without sex, so why do we diminish its role in our lives? The pleasure of the senses is literally necessary for life, so why not enjoy that and learn how to act upon those desires in both a free and moral way.

Beyond the sexual nature of the Kama Sutra, it also is a guide that teaches us how to live a good life in general. It goes in-depth on topics such as the arts, music, and literature, as well as how to be a good husband or wife.

It discusses financial matters, matters of the home, and even how to properly select a spouse that is balanced with you. It goes into great detail about how you should bathe and groom yourself, where you can meet people, and how to enjoy your day and please your spouse.

From a philosophical viewpoint, it teaches us that both men and women should engage in sensual pleasures, and that sex is not just for men to get off with. Unlike many historical texts that downplay a woman's sexual desires, the Kama Sutra takes a deep look at what a woman's sexual nature is and how to properly satisfy it both before sex as well as during.

That isn't to say, however, that the Kama Sutra is an extremely liberal book or that it holds men and women in the same regard. It is written during a time of caste systems and where women's role in a marriage was not as high as that of the man.

Men were still considered the head of the household, and much of what is described revolves around a man pursuing a woman. But, compared with other forms of literature, it does take a more liberal view of women's sexuality, as well as homosexual relationships, and the idea of having sex solely for pleasure and outside of marriage.

How to Use the Kama Sutra?

The Kama Sutra can be used in two ways, both as a practical guide as well as a philosophical work of art. Some may approach the Kama Sutra only as a guide to sex positions, and this is perfectly acceptable as a large chunk of text is dedicated to this pursuit.

However, to use the Kama Sutra fully, you must look at it as a whole and take into account both the historical significance as well as the idea that it may not be as practical as one may originally think.

Many of the sex acts described within the Kama Sutra are outside a normal person's ability and require a high degree of flexibility to perform. There are even positions within the book that are physically impossible unless the man has a very uniquely shaped lingam (penis).

Later in this book, we will look at some of the positions that are possible, however, and break down how exactly you can do them and incorporate them into your personal sex life. In many ways, there are a number of similarities between the sex acts within this book and the practice of yoga.

Through breathing as one with your partner, folding into different positions, and experiencing everything in unity, you can achieve a higher sense of awareness and satisfaction. So, even if you are unable to achieve the positions as described, think of it more like a workout for the mind and body and attempt a sexier form of yoga.

Since the positions are not always practical, you should use the Kama Sutra more as a general guide for how to deepen your pleasure. This book has taken many of the important concepts and ideas and broken them down into practical tips and advice so that you can elevate your sex life and truly engage in a more pleasurable and sensual experience.

Beyond just the sexual side of it all, the Kama Sutra should also be used as a guide on how to treat your partner both inside and outside of the bedroom. It can assist you in being more romantic and intimate, as well as teach you how to make sure your partner is satisfied completely within the relationship.

With a breakdown of different personalities and temperaments, the Kama Sutra also discusses how you can go about finding the right partner for you based on ancient concepts and ideas.

While some of the information may seem absurd in the context of today's world, not everything should be taken as a literal word. Instead, it is important that you read the Kama Sutra as a concept more than a script and that between the lines, you see that even the most ancient of dating tips are still applicable today.

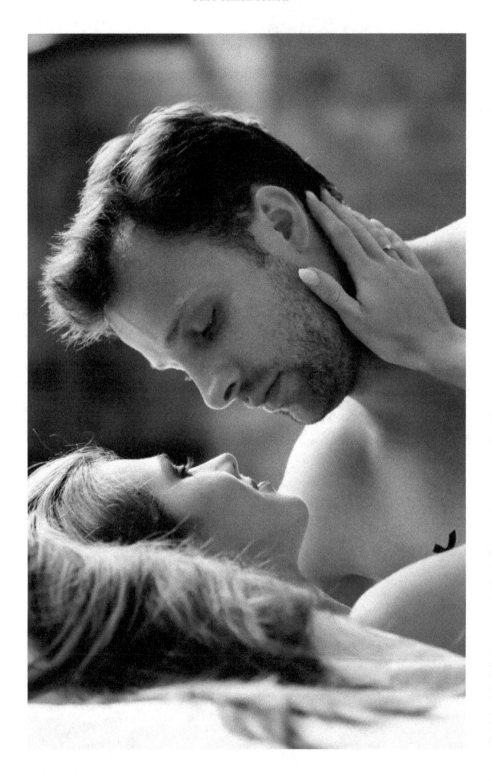

Chapter 3:

Love and the Kama Sutra

When it comes to love, there is much that can be said on how to obtain it, maintain it, and nourish it. While sex and love do not always go hand in hand, the Kama Sutra does emphasize the importance of love and goes to great lengths in order to detail exactly how a person can find love and then how they should go about ensuring that it lasts for a lifetime.

Love begins with oneself, and only then can it be extended beyond that and onto someone else. That is why the Kama Sutra makes sure to include ways to enhance your own inner love and desire but focusing on self-care and self-adornment.

The more you love yourself, the more you can love others, and the more they can love you in return. If you are down on yourself, lack self-worth, or generally feel unlovable, then you will project that onto everyone that you come in contact with.

You need to be able to present the best version of yourself possible, and always remember, there is nothing sexier in life than confidence!

Love is an extremely complex concept, and while we all may feel we understand what love is, if you ask 100 individuals to define love, you will end up with 100 different responses.

Love is defined as the feeling of attraction and desire that one feels towards another, but if you have ever been in love, you will know that it extends far beyond that shallow explanation.

Love and lust can often be confused with one another, since both play on attraction and desire, but the simplest way to break the two apart is to see love as something that is long-term, whereas lust oftentimes will fade or develop into love. When it comes to love, there are many factors that go into both falling in love, as well as staying in love with someone.

Love is not easy, nor is it free from work, and in order to maintain a healthy, loving relationship, you must be willing to sacrifice, compromise, and put in effort daily. Love is something that can grow and deepen with time like a tree grows its roots down into the earth.

What begins as only a small sapling can eventually turn into a mighty oak that even the worst of storms cannot damage. But how does one grow that tree of love? And how does one nurture it so that it is not cut down with time?

What the Kama Sutra Says About Love

The Kama Sutra discusses love in-depth and focuses heavily on marriages as the best type of union. With that said, however, it does acknowledge that not all sexual relations happen within the confines of marriage, and it does discuss the varying types of relationships that can occur.

There is even a full chapter dedicated to adultery, although the author does not necessarily condone such actions.

It is understood that love can strike at any time, with any person, and whether you are married to that individual or not, does not always matter. That is why the Kama Sutra ensures that all aspects of love are covered so that it can be applicable to all situations and types of individuals.

One part of the Kama Sutra that is important to take note of, is the fact that the author makes sure to point out that love alone is not enough to sustain a relationship, nor is it enough to make a person happy within their life.

While love is an important part of pleasure and being satisfied, it cannot be the only thing that you rely on in order to make you happy. If you pin all of your hopes and expectations onto one person, you are going to find yourself let down and dissatisfied, as one person cannot possibly meet all of your needs and desires.

Instead, you should look at love as one piece of the puzzle that is fitted with other aspects in order to create a beautiful image.

From a historical perspective, the concept of monogamy was not as enforced as it is in today's society, and instead, there were many courtesans, or prostitutes, that were utilized without judgment.

The Kama Sutra makes many notes towards courtesans, as their role in providing the ultimate sexual pleasure was very important even though it may not have involved love.

Since this isn't as applicable in today's world, however, we can adapt these teachings as more of a personal guide on how to behave. The reason why courtesans were so desirable is because they were generous lovers who focused on their partner's pleasure and had qualities about that that made them engaging and entertaining.

While you should never be something you are not just to please someone else, the idea of working on your own personality and qualities to enhance them and make yourself more interesting is certainly not a negative.

We should all work towards building up who we are, being confident in ourselves, and feeling free enough to express our innermost desires.

Physical Attraction and Love

Although love requires much more than a simple physical attraction, the way a person looks is oftentimes the first thing that draws us to them.

When you are looking to meet someone, and you know nothing about them as a person, you are going solely off of how they look to you.

If someone is physically unattractive in your eyes, there is very little chance that you will want to pursue something intimate with them, and thus the road to love is cut short.

The Kama Sutra acknowledges this and spends a lot of time discussing how to make yourself more physically desirable so that you can ultimately find love.

We are in no way suggesting that your appearance is the only thing about you that matters, but we are saying that you should pamper and care for yourself in order to be the best version of yourself that you can be.

From good hygiene practices to wearing your favorite sexy dress, making yourself look good will also make you feel good, and that creates an energy that will draw someone to you.

Different Types of Love

The Kama Sutra breaks down four different types of love, which are:

- Continual Habit

- Imagination

- Belief

- Perception of External Objects

These four types of love are not necessarily limited to just within a relationship, and they can be extended to other aspects of life as well. Below will we break down these different forms of love, discuss how they relate to your personal love life, and even give advice on how to create, maintain, and nourish each type.

Love by Continual Habit

Love by continual habit is described in the Kama Sutra as the love that comes from repetition and practice of an act. In a non-romantic way, this is the love that may develop for a certain hobby as you continue to practice it and get better at it.

The more you engage yourself and learn, the more you develop a love and passion. In a romantic way, this is the love that develops over long periods of time with an individual, either within or outside of a romantic relationship.

For example, some people may begin as friends long before they become lovers. Over time, as they do activities together, engage in long, deep talks, and grow as people they eventually fall in love. This is the continual habit of being around someone and continuing to learn about them and grow together as a couple.

This is a very strong form of love, as there is a great foundation to it, and it is built not on lust but completely on love.

This is also part of what forms the love between two individuals who have been together for many years. Over the years, that initial sexual attraction may begin to fade, and the lust that drew you together will start to become more of a slow-burning flame that keeps you both going.

It is at this point that continual habit starts to strengthen and create the love between two people, as you live together and work together you practice the art of being in love. Falling in love is not the end; it is only the beginning, and over the years you will need to continuously work on that love and nurture it so that it continues to grow.

Like blowing life into a fire, you are responsible for ensuring that the flame does not burn out.

Love by continual habit should also be extended to the individual, separate from any type of relationship. You should continuously work on learning to love yourself, showering yourself with affection, and strengthening those emotions within yourself.

Make yourself into the partner that you so desire, so that whether or not you find that person, you already know you have that completely on your own. If you can meet your own needs, satisfy yourself, and be happy when alone, then a partner is simply the icing on the cake instead of the entire cake itself.

This goes a long way in later creating healthy relationships with healthy boundaries because instead of feeling dependent on another person, you can simply enjoy being with them.

So, how do you create, maintain, and nourish love by continual habit?

- Actively spend time with the person you love or want to be in love with

- Practice being emotionally vulnerable with your partner

- Frequently touch your partner each day

- Take time each day to look in the mirror and appreciate something about yourself

- Share and create memories together

- Develop an idea of the future that you both would like to work towards

- Engage in sex frequently

These are only a very few of the ways in which you can create love via continual habit, and how you choose to do so is a completely personal choice.

What is important is not how you do it, but more so doing it in a way that creates happiness and joy in both you and your partner. It is about building and growing together and working at love every day through the practice of making it into a habit.

Love by Imagination

Love by imagination is in complete contrast to love by continual habit, as it is far from physical and exists purely within the mind. This is the type of love that has no bearing in the real world and instead is created within a fantasy of your choosing.

An innate type of love, it is one that already exists within you and requires no effort or forming of habits in order to induce. It is a type of love that exists before your partner and will continue to exist despite your partner as it is not created by them.

It can, however, be influenced and informed by your partner, but for the most part, it is simply an innate feeling that you have.

To break this down in more practical terms, we can start by looking at this love in non-romantic ways. Love by imagination is the way you love scary movies or your love for dogs over cats. It's your love for sweet treats, spicy foods, or taking walks in nature.

It's the love you feel when you think about your favorite book or movie, or when you ponder your future and all the things you will accomplish. As you can see, this type of love requires no effort and does not exist because you have worked on it.

Instead, it is a love that is easy, effortless, and oftentimes cannot be changed. You can, however, alter this type of love as you age and grow, and different experiences will shape and guide our love by imagination.

When you are young, you may hate spicy foods, but as your taste buds mature you then find yourself with a passion for the heat. This requires no effort on your part, however, it does change and grow over time.

In a romantic sense, this is the type of love that exists even before you find your partner. Your personal preference in appearance, your desire for someone funny or smart, your different viewpoints and religions, and all those other points that you think of in your head are all part of your imagination.

If you close your eyes and visualize your ideal partner, you have loved by imagination. Now, this type of love helps guide us towards the correct person for us, but it can also be a hindrance to finding a partner. In some ways, when you fall in love with the idea of someone, you set yourself up for failure.

No person is perfect, and there is no one on the planet that will check every box or meet every criterion when it comes to your imaginative person. It is very important that you remember this, as those who seek to find perfection will instead only find loneliness. What you should do is use that love by imagination to guide you towards someone, without the expectation that they will live up to every item on the list. When you use love by imagination to guide you, you go into the relationship with a base of love already there.

You know that you love people who have a great sense of humor, so you end up already loving that about your partner. If you know that you love someone who is fiercely intelligent, find a partner who is, and you will truly love that about them.

So, what are some ways in which you can create this type of love and maintain it in the long-term?

- Take the time to get inside your own head and find the qualities that are more important to you.

- Always remember that no one is perfect, and find perfection within the imperfections.

- Seek out people who match your own morals and standards.

- Engage in activities you have a pre-existing love for.

- Try out new things to find other activities you love.

- Nurture your own interests.

- Make meditation a part of your daily routine.

Remember, this type of love is innate and is not something you can create over time. Take this as more of a starter love, one which draws you to someone and begins that relationship, rather than something used to maintain it over time.

While finding someone with the right qualities will help ensure that you remain attracted long-term, it cannot sustain itself unless you strengthen and deepen that love in other ways as well.

Love from Belief

Love from belief is a love that is understood by both parties and is something felt deep within ourselves. It is the type of love in which we have no questions, no doubts, and no fears.

When we truly believe in love, when we believe in our feelings, we know that it is true and real. This is one of the strongest forms of love, and it is the one in which meaningful relationships are built upon. Love from belief stems from great communication, high levels of trust, and mutual understanding that you both have developed with time and care. It stems from years of work, as well as effort and actions purposely used to create it.

When we discuss love from belief in a non-romantic setting, we refer to things like the love a parent feels for a child or the love a person feels for a pet.

It can also include the love you feel towards your personal accomplishments or achievements, as well as the love that exists within someone's religious beliefs.

When you can feel an unwavering love and devotion, then you know you have love from belief. You are certain and sure of that love; there is no question in your mind that it is real and that you are secure within.

For romantic relationships, this is the love that lasts a lifetime. When you and your partner can look into each other's eyes and see nothing buy love reflected back, then you know that you have love from belief.

You both believe to your very core that you love the other person and that they love you in return. You are certain that they have no malicious intent, that their reasons are pure, and that their heartbeats only for you. If you are fully your partners, and they are fully yours, then you are experiencing this form of love and you will feel safe and at home within it. But this love is not without work and effort, and in order to develop it, you need to both prove your trustworthiness and have it proven to you by your spouse.

High levels of communication are required so that you are both on the same page and there are no doubts or questions left between you. Trust must be both created and never broken, for if it is ever to be broken, then love by belief will cease to exist.

Some of the ways you can develop this type of love and maintain it are:

- Avoid keeping secrets within a relationship and instead, have an air of transparency.

- Talk with your partner daily about both random topics as well as deep, important topics.

- Gaze into each other's eyes and feel their love looking back at you.

- Make sex intimate and sensual so that you feel a connection and closeness.

- Allow yourself to be vulnerable with your partner

- Lean on your partner in times of need, and allow them to lean on you in return.

- Make the effort to cultivate your love by having special date nights.

Much of this love stems from a trust within yourself and deep knowledge, so it is important you are in tune with your own feelings and intuitions. It is only by being open to this kind of love that you will ever receive it, and if your heart is closed off, then you can never experience love by belief.

Love Created from the Perception of External Objects

Within the Kama Sutra, this is considered the highest form of love, and all other forms of love are there only to lead to and enhance this. This is the love you feel for what is in front of you, and it is a tangible form of love based upon what you can see and feel.

All of the forms we discussed above are based on this, as each is used as a way to feel, show, and create love for that which is external to yourself. How you see something and experience, it is going to create and shape your love for it, and without an external source, there honestly is nothing to actually love.

When you look upon your favorite item, or a close friend, or even a family member, you will immediately feel a sense of love. This comes from the love that already exists, created by habit or by imagination, it does not matter.

No matter how you created that love, it exists, and the simple sight of the object ignites those feelings and makes you happy. Most commonly thought of when people think about love, this is what we are all most familiar with, and it is the simplest form of love for people to understand. It requires no deeper thought and no effort on our part, and instead is a natural reaction to everything else that goes on behind the scene.

When your dog looks at you with nothing but love in their eyes, it is not because they have worked at it or are thinking it over and analyzing it. Instead, they see you and their brain lights up, and they feel that true love.

That is a true example of love created from the perception of external objects, as it is simply the sight of you that makes the dog feel so much love.

In romantic relationships, this is the love you feel when you look over at your partner throughout the day, or when you wake up in the morning to their face. There are no second thoughts, nor do you analyze why you feel and react the way you do. Instead, it feels incredibly natural and right. This is the kind of love we need the most, and it doesn't matter how you went about creating it.

Whether you started off as friends and built it via habit, or you imagined your dream spouse and found someone who checked off a lot of those boxes, none of that even crosses your mind when you look upon them.

Instead, it comes down to how you perceive them, and that your mind associates them with something positive and worthwhile. As you interact with them, you feel love. As you laugh together, you feel happiness towards each other. As you cry in each other's arms, you feel safe.

All of this is external displays of the love you feel inside, and it is the most important form of love as it reaffirms everything we think and feel inside.

So, if this love is completely external, how do we go about creating it and nourishing it?

- Spend quality time with your partner so that you are engaged in activities together.

- Allow yourself to simply experience love without analyzing it.

- Cuddle in bed and hold each other without any expectations.

- Physically touch your partner often.

- Hold hands when you are out walking around.

- Kiss each morning before you leave for work.

- Smile when you see your partner so that they get a visual representation of your love for them.

The four types of love are not mutually exclusive, and instead should be viewed as equally important in creating and maintain a healthy, long term relationship. All aspects of love need to be there in order to make it last, so ensure that you are creating daily habits as well as seeking a partner who fulfills your greatest desires.

Believe in your partner, trust them, and never give them a reason to doubt how you honestly feel about them, so that you both can fully believe in what you have together. And beyond all of that, simply exist within that love and interact with every day. You don't always need to be analyzing every thought and feeling, as being in the moment can be much more satisfying.

How to Find a Spouse

One area that the Kama Sutra goes very in-depth, is how to go about finding a spouse for yourself. There are a number of different sections that discuss this matter, and each provides practical tips to assist you.

Some of the advice given may not be as applicable in today's world, as the invention of the internet has changed the dating landscape significantly.

Also, many of us date for pleasure and not always with the goal of marriage, so this may not apply to everyone who is reading it. However, marriage was an important aspect of life back when the Kama Sutra was written, so it should come as no surprise that much of the book is written with married couples in mind.

In the Kama Sutra, discussion about marriage begins with finding someone within the same caste as you, and nowadays, this is not nearly as relevant.

In modern times we avoid breaking people down into different caste systems, but there is some truth with regards to finding someone of a similar background.

You want to ensure that you and your partner have similar beliefs and morals, as individuals who are too strongly opposed to the others' ideas may not work out in the long-term. This is especially important when it comes to key points, such as:

- Do you and your partner both want children?

- How do you plan on raising those children?

- Are you devout in your religious beliefs?

- What are the ideas of gender roles within a marriage?

- Are your political beliefs similar?

- How do you feel towards alcohol and drugs?

- Are your sex drives similar?

- Do you both want to get married?

- How do you approach financial matters?

- What do you expect from a partner?

- Where do you see yourself living?

- What are your main goals in life?

While a difference in opinion can be healthy and is even encouraged, if you differ on vital points then you are doomed to fail. If one of you dreams of being a parent, but the other is absolutely against having children, there will eventually be resentment between you as one partner will feel that a core desire is not being met.

With regards to the Kama Sutra, the majority of the text on marriage discusses how a man should go about finding a wife and what he should look for in the woman that he marries.

There is also a lot of discussion regarding marriages in which the man has multiple wives, and the role each wife should take in the relationship. This information is not as applicable today, so we have opted to leave it out of this chapter. But in order to properly cover everything that exists within the Kama Sutra, it is still worth mentioning that it exists.

How one seeks out a wife is not the only thing that is discussed, and its fact the Kama Sutra goes into great detail regarding how a man should then pursue a woman and win her over.

We will discuss the courtship aspect of this much deeper in chapter 3, but for now, we will simply look at what a man should be looking for. The Kama Sutra mentions the following in terms of what a man should avoid when looking for a wife:

- A man should not marry a woman who is asleep or crying.

- He should not try and marry a woman who is already married.

- He should avoid someone with a bad sounding name, or whose name ends in the letter R or L.

- A man should not marry a woman who is disfigured, has crooked thighs, or is bald.

- He should seek to marry a virgin who has reached puberty.

- A man should not marry his friend or his sister.

What we can take away from the above list is that times certainly have changed, and many of what is listed seems both childish and absurd by today's standards.

However, some points, such as not marrying someone who is asleep or who is crying, are still very much valid and should be respected and adhered to! So, what should an ideal bride be?

- She should be beautiful to look upon.

- She should come from a good family.

- Her age should be three years or younger than the man.

- She should be wealthy.

- Her body should be in good health and have lucky marks on it.

- She should not have been married previously.

- Most importantly, she should be the one that the man loves.

Now, that last point may seem contradictory to the others, for what if the man falls in love with a woman that is bald? Or a woman that is not three years younger than himself?

Well, it is said in the Kama Sutra that above all else, the only that thing that will bring true happiness and prosperity is marrying someone that you are attached to and to whom you feel love. Without love, there is no reason to marry, and this is something we can attest to even today.

There are different types of marriages discussed within the Kama Sutra, but the main type is what is called Gandharva marriage. This is the type of marriage when two people are equally attracted to one another, and without any interference from others consent to be married.

There are no rituals or family involved, and instead is private between the two who are to be wed. While this was seen as not socially correct, it is the type of marriage that is brought about due solely to love, and this is one of the highest forms of marriage attainable.

What we can take from the Kama Sutra in terms of marriage is that love should be the basis for a successful marriage.

Regardless of what your spouse looks like or what family they are born into, if you love the person, you should seek them out and create that relationship with them. Looks will eventually fade, and social status can change, but what should be everlasting is the love you have for one another. As long as you have that, the marriage is starting out on the right foot.

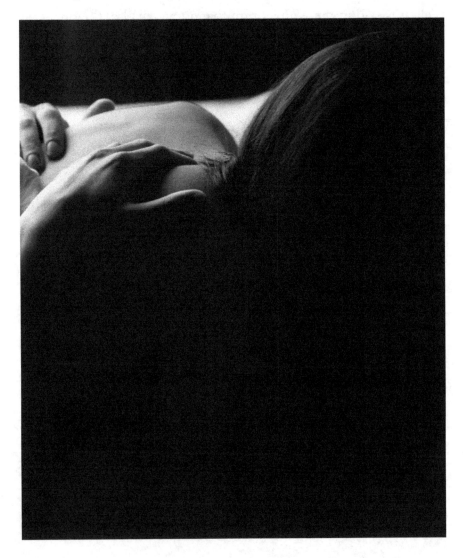

Chapter 4:

Flirting and Courtship

Flirting and courtship are two very important aspects of any relationship, as without them we would never be able to woo our partner and attract them to us.

We all have our own unique style of flirting, some of us being better at it than others, but thankfully the Kama Sutra lays out exactly what we should be doing in order to be the best flirter possible.

Before we dive into the art of courtship and the tricks to up your flirting game, we will break down exactly what flirting and courtship are and how they differ. Flirting is something that is done with a less serious intention in mind than when you court someone.

Flirting can be both sexual as well as friendly, and people can engage in it for fun just as much as they can use it to attract a partner. Typically flirting involves using both verbal and non-verbal communication in order to let someone know that you are interested in them. It can involve a wink, touching someone's arm, laughing at their jokes, or any other of ways in which you showcase your interest.

Courting, on the other hand, is more serious in nature, and it is dating someone with the intention of marrying them. Some religious beliefs feel that the only acceptable form of dating is courting, while others engage in courting, not for religious reasons but because they are simply at a point in life where they are looking to get married.

Courting can, and should, involve flirting, but it is used to win the other person over and entice them to want to marry you. It is never simply used to instigate a fling or sexual encounter, as that would be in direct contradiction to the point of courting.

Now that we have a basic understanding of the two terms, what exactly does the Kama Sutra say when it comes to courting and flirting?

Meeting the Person, You Want to Date

To begin with, the Kama Sutra starts by mentioning that anyone looking to court another should be realistic in their approach.

What this means is that any quality that they are seeking in another, they should possess that quality themselves; otherwise, they have no right to expect it of their partner.

For instance, if you want your partner to be extremely good looking, you should also be extremely good looking; otherwise, you should not put such a demand on someone else. Once you have your expectations in check, then you can begin the processes of searching for your partner.

So, how does one go about seeking out a woman in ancient times when there was no social media and no dating apps? Well, the Kama Sutra suggests the following ways:

- A woman who is ready to be married should be dressed up nicely by her family and placed in a location where she can be seen.

- Women seeking a husband should attend events such as sporting matches and marriage ceremonies.

- Men should throw parties in which games are played, causing everyone to interact with each other.

- Through friendships, two people can then meet and get to know each other.

- By asking their parents, a man can have a wife arranged for him.

Of course, we can add much more to this list for current times, so if you are at the point in your life where you are looking to meet someone and build towards marriage, or a future in general, you can try the following more common suggestions as well:

- **Try going online and joining a dating site** - Nowadays there are numerous different sites, all catering to different individuals and desires, so you are likely to find a site that is perfect for you and finding a partner that matches what you are after.

- **Ask your friends to hook you up with someone** - We know the idea of going on a blind date sounds terrifying, but your friends do know you well, so there is always the chance that they might know someone who fits in with what you are looking for.

- **Participate in a sport or hobby** – Take up a new activity that interests you in order to meet new people and also meet someone who shares similar interests with you. Not only will you already have something to talk about, but it gets you out of the house and on a mini-date right from day one.

- **Take the bus to work** – While your morning commute is never fun, why not turn it into an opportunity to meet someone? Public transportation puts you in close proximity with new people that you have never met before.

However, you choose to approach meeting someone, that is only the first step in courtship, as the real work is what comes afterward.

Beginning a Courtship

Once you have found an individual who interests you, who you would like to get closer with, and possibly start a relationship, how are you supposed to let them know that you are interested?

In modern times, we have many ways of determining if someone is interested in us, and many of these various ways full under the heading of flirting.

When we are attracted to someone, either physically or mentally, or both, our bodies automatically respond to them in specific ways. Some of what we do is deliberate, while other actions are completely subconscious and are naturally done simply because we want to be near someone.

Some of the common ways of flirting that you may be more familiar with are:

- Making direct eye contact.

- Holding eye contact longer than normal.

- Smiling when you look at a person.

- Touching them on the arm when you talk.

- Winking from across a room.

- Complimenting the other person.

- Biting of the lip.

- Playing with your hair.

- Mirroring another person's movements.

- Laugh at their silly jokes.

- Stand closely.

- Stare at their lips.

- Keep your arms uncrossed and open.

- Tease them playfully.

- Drop a witty pick-up line.

- Send a flirtatious text message.

Sadly, you won't find any of these located within the Kama Sutra as back in ancient India, flirting and courting were done much differently. To compare with the above list, let's take a look at different ways in which the Kama Sutra suggests a man flirts with a woman to show her that he is interested and to engage her attention:

- Spend time with her and entertain her with games.

- Pick flowers and turn them into a garland.

- Cook meals together.

- Play with dice or cards.

- Playgroup games such as hide and seek.

- Do gymnastic exercises together.

- Show kindness to her friends.

- Partake in services for her maid's daughter to win her over.

- Get her gifts that no other girls have.

- Give her handmade dolls and wooden figures.

- Create temples for her dedicated to different goddesses.

- Make her see him as someone who can do everything for her.

- Meet her in private.

- Tell her exciting stories.

- Perform tricks and juggle.

- Sing for her and take her to festivals.

- Give her flowers and jewelry.

- Teach her nurses daughter the 64 forms of pleasure.

While many of these sounds a bit strange in today's time, there is a lot we can take away from this list.

Mainly, everything described above is meant to make the man stand out from other men that may have an interest in the same woman.

This is exactly what modern-day flirting and courting involves as well, as you want to make the other person see what you have to offer and what they will find in you that they cannot find in someone else.

Flirting and courting are meant to entice another person, that is their sole purpose, and to let that person know that you would like to be in a relationship with them, or at the very least engage in some sort of romantic endeavor.

Many people get stressed out by the idea of flirting, and so often, you will hear individuals remark that they are unable to flirt or are the worst at doing so.

This is simply a false idea that they have gotten into them hear, and they are making it into something much more complicated than it needs to be.

Flirting does not need to be anything more than smiling at a person you like or going out of your way to do something nice for them. All you are aiming to do is make them feel special and noticed, and to hopefully get them to notice you in return.

The best way to go about it if you lack confidence is to simply start off small. You don't need to perform a magic trick or juggle, and instead, you can simply compliment their outfit or send them a text asking about their day.

The basic act of taking notice goes a very long way as it shows the person you are thinking of them and that you are interested in who they are.

Don't overcomplicate things, and let it progress naturally as you feel more comfortable. Once you get outside of your own head, you will find flirting to be one of the most natural acts possible.

A Woman's State of Mind

Within the Kama Sutra, Vatsyayana goes into detail about a woman's state of mind during flirting and courtship and breaks down the different ways she may feel and react, as well as how many should respond to her.

Some of the advice is practical and useful even in today's world, but other tips are much more non-consensual and should not ever be utilized. Here are the mindsets that are mentioned along with the details attributed to each one:

A Woman Who Listens but Does Not Show Any Interest

In this scenario, a man should attempt to persuade her by using a middle man instead of just doing it on his own. A good option would be her nurse's daughter or one of her friends.

If a Woman Meets a Man Once and Then the Next Time Is Better Dressed

This indicates that she is very interested, and thus the man will need to do little in order to win her over. If, however, after a long period of time she still does not consent to be with him, then he should be wary but still keep her as a close friend.

When a Woman Avoids A Man Out of Respect

In this scenario, it will be difficult to win her over, but the man can do so by keeping her as a close friend and also employing the assistance of a very crafty middle man.

If a Woman Turns a Man Down Harshly

When this happens, a man should abandon his attempts to win her over and move on to someone else, for she had no interest in anything he has to offer her.

When Meeting Privately, She Allows His Touch but Pretends Not to Notice

If this happens, then it means she is interested but playing coy, so he should continue on with his advances. It will require extra patience, but he can begin by putting his arm around her while she sleeps and seeing how she reacts. If it is a favorable reaction, then he can continue on by drawing her closer to him and continuing on from there.

If a Woman Does Not Encourage nor Discourage a Man's Advances but Instead Is Hidden Away in a Place He Cannot Get To

The only option in this situation is to employ the help of someone who is close to her in order to communicate his advances. The best option would be the daughter of her maid.

If the woman does not respond to the man through the go-between, then he should reconsider whether or not to continue pursuing her.

When A Woman Proclaims Her Own Interest in The Man

If this happens, then the man can know for sure that she wants to be with him, and he can delight in enjoying her fully. In order to realize this situation, however, the man must know the ways in which a woman will show her interest. Ways in which a woman will manifest her love towards a man are:

- She speaks to him without being addressed first.

- She meets with him in private.

- When she talks her voice trembles.

- Her hands and feet will perspire.

- Her face will blush with delight.

- She will shampoo his body and rub his head.

- When washing him she only uses one hand, and instead uses the other hand to caress him.

- She stands motionless with both hands pressed against him.

- She bends down and places her face on his thighs.

- If she places her hand upon him, she keeps it there for a long period of time.

The most important thing noted when discussing wooing over a woman, however, is how she responds within the first conversation that a man has with her.

The Kama Sutra notes that a man must find a way to be introduced to the woman that he is interested in, and from there, he can then carry out a conversation to assess her feelings. By subtle means of flirting, he should try and let the woman know that he has love for her, and if she responds to this in a positive way, then he should continue on with pursuing her over time.

If the woman is very open to his expressions of love, and outwardly responds in a favorable manner, then he knows he will be able to gain her over as a wife very easily. Finally, if a woman is open enough to express her love back verbally, then the man will know right then and there that she is his.

Vatsyayana believed that this was true for all women, regardless of who they are, where they were from, or how they were raised, and in many ways, this still holds true today.

It may all sound like very obvious information, but when our brains are overtaken by feelings of love, our judgment can become clouded, and we may miss some of the most obvious signals that someone else is attracted to us as well.

That is why it is important to have them written down in a book like the Kama Sutra, so that even in moments of overwhelming desire, we are reminded of the simple truths that come with flirting and courting. Mainly, what we are discussing are various aspects of consent, and how pursuing someone who is not interested in us will not get us very far. While the Kama Sutra often encourages a man to keep trying, it specifies that when a woman harshly turns you down, then it is time to leave her be.

You should never force yourself on someone else, and in fact, why would you want to? We all want to be loved and desired, and none of us should settle for someone who dislikes us or isn't as invested as we are in them.

While the Kama Sutra may have some outdated views on flirting and courtship, the basic principles are still applicable even after all of the centuries which have passed since it was written. Take the time to show someone you are interested, go the extra mile, make them laugh, and employ the help of a mutual friend if you are shy are unsure. Whatever you choose to do, make sure you enjoy the process as flirting and courting are almost sport like in their nature.

This is when new feelings are blossoming, and a different picture of the future will unfold in your mind. The best thing you can do is to lose yourself in those feelings and to simply see where they take you. Not every person you pursue will work out, but eventually, you will find that one person that appreciates what you have to offer and will offer you just as much in return.

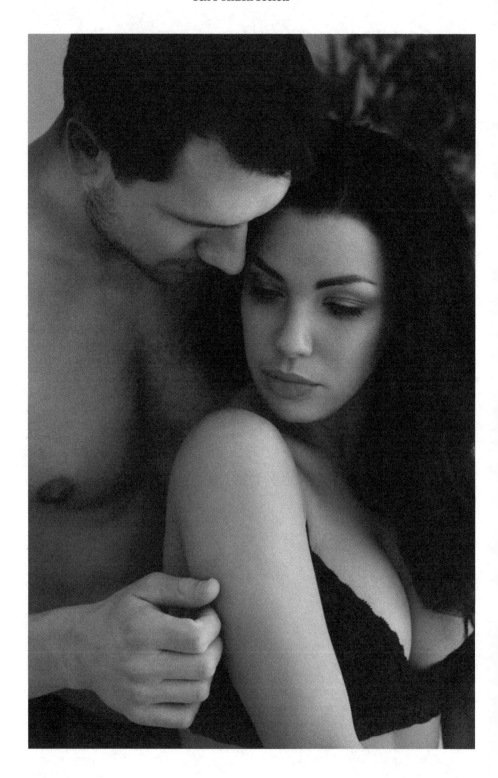

Conclusion

J ust because you've finished this book doesn't mean there is nothing left to learn on the topic, expanding your horizons is the only way to find the mastery you seek.

It is your sole responsibility to internalize and practice your key take always for ultimate results.

You may need to break down important points and prioritize them for easy and coordinated steps to action. Once you decide to try out some of the practices discussed to ensure you understand that your partner's consent is of utmost importance as it is a critical determinant in the acquisition of pleasure and stimulation.

Start with the easy sex positions as you work your way up through intermediate ones and, eventually, the advanced positions. A significant first step in making sexual stimulation should be through seduction, which expresses your swish to make sexual advances.

Keep in mind that it can be hard to circumvent a partner who is unwilling to try out new sex positions or explore additional sex variants. Therefore, you should approach them with respect and love and persuade them of the need for trying out something different, and it may be a step to indulge in an ecstasy of sexual stimulation and orgasm.

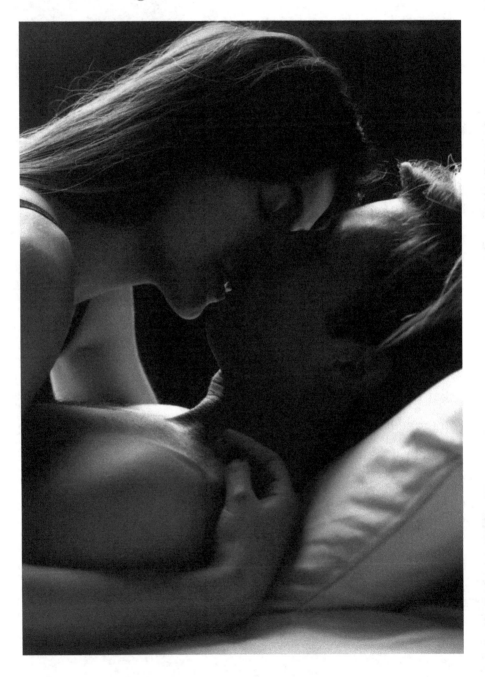

CPSIA information can be obtained
at www.ICGtesting.com
Printed in the USA
BVHW091051230621
610290BV00010B/171